The Ultimate Lean And Green Cookbook For Beginners

A Superlative Guide To Understanding The Concepts Days Fueling Hacks & Lean And Green Recipes To Help You Keep Healthy And Lose Weight By Harnessing The Power Of Fuelings

Lisa G. Torres

Table of Contents

Introduction

I f you are looking to lose weight fast and you don't always have enough time to cook, this regimen is the best option for you. However, this diet program requires that you work with a coach on a one-on-one guide and counseling. It includes branded products known as Fuelings and homemade food known as Lean & Green meals.

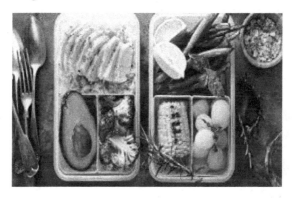

These Fuelings have over 60 products that are low in carb and high in protein. They have probiotic cultures with health-promoting bacteria that boost gut health. Some of them are bars, shakes, cereals, cookies, pasta, puddings, etc.

The Diet Programs

The program has three versions, which include 2 weight loss plans and a maintenance plan.

- **Optimal Weight 5&1**: This plan is the most popular among the program plans. It is made up of daily 5 Fuelings and 1 lean and green meal.

- **Optimal Weight 4&2&1**: If you need more calories, this plan is for you. It is more flexible and includes 4 Fuelings, 2 lean and green, and 1 snack every day.

- **Optimal Health 3&3**: With 3 Fuelings and 3 lean and green meals, it is designed to help in weight maintenance.

Diet Guide

For a quick weight loss goal, the Optimal Weight 5&1 Plan may be the best plan to start with. Most people with the target of losing weight usually go for this plan as it helps them to drop up to 12 pounds within 12 weeks.

In the Optimal Weight 5&1 Plan, you are expected to eat one lean and green meal and five Fuelings. These meals are to be eaten every 2-3 hours intervals. Then, you will back it up with 30 minutes of exercise. Your coach will direct you on the best approach.

However, the daily carbs from meals and Fuelings should not exceed 100 grams. You can get meals and Fuelings from the company. Though it may not be cost-effective, this book is designed to help you save costs. You can prepare the meals by yourself to reduce costs.

There are a plethora of recipes in this book to help you along the process for your daily meals. You can also eat out, but keep in mind that you must follow the diet plan as instructed by your coach. However, alcohol is highly restricted for this plan.

Once you get to your desired weight, you are expected to enter the maintenance phase. This is a transition phase that requires a gradual increase in your daily calorie intake to no more than 1,550 cal. You can add a wider variety of food to your daily meals, which include fruits, whole grains, and low-fat dairy.

The maintenance phase is expected to last for 6 weeks before you move to the Optimal Health 3&3 Plan. In this plan, your daily food intake will be 3 Fuelings and 3 lean and green meals.

In this diet, most people that follow the diet usually opt for the 5&1 plan. The 5&1 program is made up of 5 Fuelings and 1 high protein low-carb meal. There are over 60 fueling options in this diet, and these options include bars, puddings, shakes, soups, biscuits, etc. These Fuelings contain probiotics that help to promote digestive health.

The interesting aspect of this diet is its flexibility, which makes it easier to work with. Once you reach your desired weight goal, you can easily switch to the 3&3 plan. Transitioning to this weight-maintenance plan is easy since you have already changed the old unhealthy eating habits. For those looking to consume more calories, the 4&2&1 plan is your best bet. With the 4&2&1 plan, you take 4 Fuelings, 2 healthy lean and green meals, and 1 snack.

How This Diet Can Help You Lose Weight

How much weight you lose on the this diet depends mostly on how active and how you follow the plan. If you stick with the plan and stay very active, you will lose more weight. Many have tried it, and it worked perfectly well. The following research studies show how effective the diet can be when strictly followed. Though the research is mostly on Medifast, this diet and Medifast have identical macro-nutrients and can be interchanged to achieve the same result. So, the studies are valid for both this diet and Medifast plans.

- A study published in the Obesity journal in 2016 showed that after 12 weeks of observing the diet guides, obese people lost 8.8% body weight.

- The study released by John Hopkins Medicine that ran for 12 weeks revealed that weight-loss programs like Medifast are effective for a long-term weight loss goal.

- A study in the Nutrition Journal carried out in 2015 shows that 310 obese and overweight people who followed the diet plans lost 24 lb in 12 weeks. In the 24th week, the average weight loss recorded was 35 lb.

- Another study published in the Nutrition Journal shows that 90 obese adults who followed the 5&1 plan lost an average of 30 pounds in 16 weeks.

- The analysis published in the Eating and Weight Disorder Journal in 2008 shows that the average weight loss recorded on

324 obese patients in 12 weeks was 21 lb and 26 ½ lb after 24 weeks. However, these patients also took appetite suppressant.

Is Diet Easy To Follow?

If you are someone like me that likes trying so many treats and yummy recipes almost every day, the present regimen may not be easy in the long term. However, this diet is programmed to accommodate both long-term and short-term goals. There are three major diet plans to choose from to suit your desired eating habit.

The 5&1 plan may not be easy in the long-term, but there are over 60 fueling options to work with. Moreover, you have a plethora of resources where you can get recipes, including this cookbook with so many mouthwatering recipes to make.

Unlike most weight-loss diets, you don't need to stress yourself counting calories, points, or carbs. Though they are needed for reference purposes, you don't need to kill yourself over it as long as the meals you are taking are lean and green meals.

Interestingly, you can easily eat out while on this diet. The main thing is for you to understand the guidelines and follow them judiciously. You can as well download the eating out guide from the company website to help you easily navigate the buffets and eateries.

CHAPTER 1:

What to Eat

Best Foods for LEAN and GREEN Diet

Your homemade meals are expected to be mostly low-carb vegetables, lean proteins, and a few healthy fats. Low-carb beverages such as coffee, water, tea, unsweetened almond milk, etc, are allowed, but in small amounts.

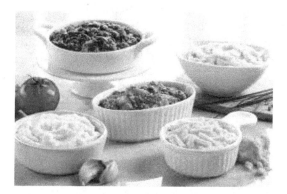

- The recommended foods for your lean and green meals are;

- Fish and Shellfish: trout, halibut, salmon, shrimp, tuna, crab, lobster, scallops.

- Meat: Lean beef, pork chop, tenderloin, turkey, chicken, lamb.

- Eggs: egg whites, whole eggs, and egg beaters.

- Soy: tofu

- Oil: vegetable oils - flaxseed, olive, canola, walnut, lemon oil, etc

- Fats: avocado, olives, almonds, pistachios, reduced-fat margarine, walnuts, etc.

- Vegetables: zucchini, cauliflower, celery, mushrooms, eggplant, pepper, spinach, cucumbers, squash, broccoli, collard, jicama, etc.

- Snacks (sugar-free): mints, popsicle, gum, gelatin, etc.

- Beverages (sugar-free): coffee, water, tea, almond milk, etc.

- Seasoning and condiments: spices, dried herbs, salsa, cocktail sauce, yellow mustard, lemon juice, soy sauce, lime juice, etc.

Avoid These Foods

Except for the carbs in the Fuelings, the present diet restricts most foods and beverages with carb content. Some fats are not allowed, including fried foods. Avoid the following foods in your daily meals;

- Refined grains: including pasta, flour tortillas, cookies, white rice, white bread, cakes, biscuits, etc.

- Whole fat dairy: including yogurt, milk, and cheese.

- Fried foods: including fish, veggies, meats, pastries, etc.

- Fats: like coconut oil, butter, etc.

- Alcohol: all types.

- Beverages: like an energy drink, fruit juice, sweet tea, soda, etc

If you are on the 5&1 plan, you need to avoid the following foods in your daily meal. You can introduce them in the transition phase;

- Starchy veggies: white potatoes, sweet potatoes, peas, and corn.

- Whole grains: brown rice, whole grain bread, whole-wheat pasta, etc.

- Low-fat dairy: cheese, yogurt, and milk.

- Legumes: beans, peas, soybeans, lentils, etc.

- Fruits: fresh fruits. Eat more berries when you enter the transition phase.

CHAPTER 2:

Lean and Green Recipes

1.   Chicken Salad

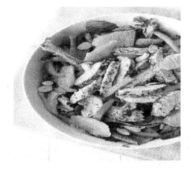

Preparation Time: 5 minutes

Cooking Time: 25 minutes

Servings: 4

Ingredients:

For Chicken:

- 1 ¾ lb. boneless, skinless chicken breast

- ¼ teaspoon each of pepper and salt (or as desired)

- 1 ½ tablespoon of butter, melted

For Mediterranean salad:

- 1 cup of sliced cucumber

- 6 cups of romaine lettuce that is torn or roughly chopped

- 10 pitted Kalamata olives

- 1 pint of cherry tomatoes

- 1/3 cup of reduced-fat feta cheese

- ¼ teaspoon each of pepper and salt (or lesser)

- 1 small lemon juice (it should be about 2 tablespoons)

Directions:

1. Preheat your oven or grill to about 350°F.

2. Season the chicken with salt, butter, and black pepper

3. Roast or grill chicken until it reaches an internal temperature of 165°F in about 25 minutes. Once your chicken breasts are cooked, remove and keep aside to rest for about 5 minutes before you slice it.

4. Combine all the salad ingredients you have and toss everything together very well

5. Serve the chicken with Mediterranean salad

Nutrition: Calories 340, Fat 4, Carbs 9, Protein 45

2.   Chipotle Chicken & Cauliflower Rice Bowls

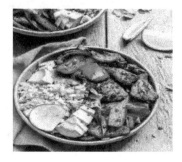

Preparation Time: 10 minutes

Cooking Time: 20 minutes

Servings: 4

Ingredients:

- 1/3 cup of salsa

- 1 quantity of 14.5 oz. of can fire-roasted diced tomatoes

- 1 canned chipotle pepper + 1 teaspoon sauce

- ½ teaspoon of dried oregano

- 1 teaspoon of cumin

- 1 ½ lb. of boneless, skinless chicken breast

- ¼ teaspoon of salt

- 1 cup of reduced-fat shredded Mexican cheese blend

- 4 cups of frozen riced cauliflower

- ½ medium-sized avocado, sliced

Directions:

1. Combine the first ingredients in a blender and blend until they become smooth

2. Place chicken inside your instant pot, and pour the sauce over it. Cover the lid and close the pressure valve. Set it to 20 minutes at high temperature. Let the pressure release on its own before

opening. Remove the piece and the chicken, and then add it

back to the sauce.

3. Microwave the riced cauliflower according to the directions on

    the package

4. Before you serve, divide the riced cauliflower, cheese, avocado,

    and chicken equally among the 4 bowls.

Nutrition: Calories 276, Fat 12, Carbs 19, Protein 35

3. Lemon Garlic Oregano Chicken with Asparagus

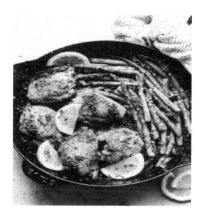

Preparation Time: 5 minutes

Cooking Time: 40 minutes

Servings: 4

Ingredients:

- 1 small lemon, juiced (this should be about 2 tablespoons of lemon juice)

- 1 ¾ lb. of bone-in, skinless chicken thighs

- 2 tablespoon of fresh oregano, minced

- 2 cloves of garlic, minced

- 2 lbs. of asparagus, trimmed

- ¼ teaspoon each or less for black pepper and salt

Directions:

1. Preheat the oven to about 350°F.

2. Put the chicken in a medium-sized bowl. Now, add the garlic, oregano, lemon juice, pepper, and salt and toss together to combine.

3. Roast the chicken in the air fryer oven until it reaches an internal temperature of 165°F in about 40 minutes. Once the chicken thighs have been cooked, remove and keep aside to rest.

4. Now, steam the asparagus on a stovetop or in a microwave to the desired doneness.

5. Serve asparagus with the roasted chicken thighs.

Nutrition: Calories 356, Fat 10, Carbs 10, Protein 24

4. **Sheet Pan Chicken Fajita Lettuce Wraps**

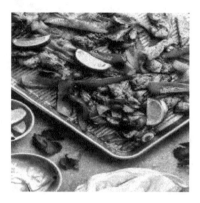

Preparation Time: 15 minutes

Cooking Time: 30 minutes

Servings: 2

Ingredients:

- 1 lb. chicken breast, thinly sliced into strips

- 2 teaspoon of olive oil

- 2 bell peppers, thinly sliced into strips

- 2 teaspoon of fajita seasoning

- 6 leaves from a romaine heart

- Juice of half a lime ¼ cup plain of non-fat Greek yogurt

Directions:

1. Preheat your oven to about 400°F

2. Combine all of the ingredients except for lettuce in a large plastic bag that can be resealed. Mix very well to coat vegetables and chicken with oil and seasoning evenly.

3. Spread the contents of the bag evenly on a foil-lined baking sheet. Bake it for about25-30 minutes, until the chicken is thoroughly cooked.

4. Serve on lettuce leaves and topped with Greek yogurt if you like

Nutrition: Calories 387, Fat 6, Carbs 14, Protein 18

CHAPTER 3:

Fuelings

5.   Avocado Bites

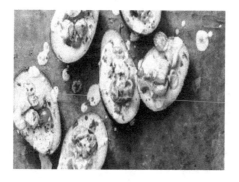

Preparation time: 10 minutes

Cooking time: 0 minutes

Servings: 2

Ingredients:

- 2 avocados, peeled, pitted, and cubed

- 2 tablespoons sweet paprika

- juice of 1 lemon

- 1 teaspoon basil, dried

- 1 teaspoon oregano, dried

- Salt and black pepper to the taste

Directions:

1. Mix the ingredients and serve.

Nutrition: calories 60, fat 3, carbs 4.2, protein 4.4

6.   Chives Dip

Preparation time: *10 minutes*

Cooking time: *0 minutes*

Servings: *4*

Ingredients:

- 2 cups chives, chopped

- 1/2 cup almond milk

- ¼ cup chopped carrot

- ¼ cup chopped red onion

- Salt and black pepper to the taste

- 1 teaspoon sweet paprika

Directions:

1. In a blender, mix the chives with the carrot and the other ingredients and blend well.

2. Divide into bowls and serve.

Nutrition: calories 210, fat 3.4, carbs 6.4, protein 6

7.   Stuffed Avocado

Preparation time: 10 minutes

Cooking time: 0 minutes

Servings: 2

Ingredients:

- 2 avocados, halved, pitted and flesh scooped out

- ¼ cup chives, chopped

- ½ cup carrot, grated

- ½ cup kale, chopped

- 1 teaspoon dried thyme

- A pinch of salt and black pepper

- ¼ teaspoon cayenne pepper

- 1 teaspoon paprika

- Salt and black pepper to the taste

- 2 tablespoons lemon juice

Directions:

1. In a bowl, mix the chives with carrots, avocado flesh, and the other ingredients except for the avocado shells and stir well.

2. Stuff the avocado skins with this mix, arrange them on a platter, and serve as an appetizer.

Nutrition: calories 160, fat 10, carbs 4,2, protein 5.5

8.   Radish Chips

Preparation time: 10 minutes

Cooking time: 20 minutes

Servings: 4

Ingredients:

- 2 teaspoons avocado oil

- 15 radishes, sliced

- A pinch of salt and black pepper

- 1 tablespoon chopped chives

Directions:

1. Arrange radish slices on a lined baking sheet, add the other ingredients, toss and place in the oven at 375 degrees F.

2. Bake for 10 minutes on each side, divide into bowls and serve

   cold.

Nutrition: calories 30, fat 1, fiber 2, carbs 7, protein 1

CHAPTER 4:

Lunch Recipes

9.   Roasted Cornish Hen

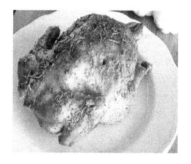

Preparation time: 15 minutes

Cooking time: 1 hour

Servings: 8

- 1 tablespoon dried basil, crushed

- 2 tablespoons lemon pepper

- 1 tablespoon poultry seasoning

- Salt, as required

- 4 (1½-pound) Cornish game hens, rinsed and dried completely

- 2 tablespoons olive oil

- 1 yellow onion, chopped

- 1 celery stalk, chopped

- 1 green bell pepper, seeded and chopped

Directions:

1. Preheat your oven to 375°F. Arrange lightly greased racks in 2 large roasting pans.

2. In a bowl, mix well basil, lemon pepper, poultry seasoning, and salt.

3. Coat each hen with oil and then rub evenly with the seasoning mixture.

4. In another bowl, mix together the onion, celery, and bell pepper.

5. Stuff the cavity of each hen loosely with veggie mixture.

6. Arrange the hens into prepared roasting pans, keeping plenty of space between them.

7. Roast for about 60 minutes or until the juices run clear.

8. Remove the hens from the oven and place them onto a cutting board.

9. With a foil piece, cover each hen loosely for about 10 minutes before carving.

10. Cut into desired size pieces and serve.

Nutrition: Calories 432, Fat 18, Carbs 4, Protein 23

10.   Butter Chicken

Preparation time: 15 minutes

Cooking time: 28 minutes

Servings: 5

Ingredients:

- 3 tablespoons unsalted butter

- 1 medium yellow onion, chopped

- 2 garlic cloves, minced

- 1 teaspoon fresh ginger, minced

- 1½ pounds grass-fed chicken breasts, cut into ¾-inch chunks

- 2 tomatoes, chopped finely

- 1 tablespoon garam masala

- 1 teaspoon red chili powder

- 1 teaspoon ground cumin

- Salt and ground black pepper, as required

- 1 cup heavy cream

- 2 tablespoons fresh cilantro, chopped

Directions:

1. Melt butter in a large wok over medium-high heat and sauté the onions for about 5–6 minutes.

2. Now, add in ginger and garlic and sauté for about 1 minute.

3. Add the tomatoes and cook for about 2–3 minutes, crushing with the back of the spoon.

4. Stir in the chicken spices, salt, and black pepper, and cook for about 6–8 minutes or until the desired doneness of the chicken.

5. Stir in the heavy cream and cook for about 8–10 more minutes, stirring occasionally.

6. Garnish with fresh cilantro and serve hot.

Nutrition: Calories 506, Fat 22, Carbs 4, Protein 32

11.   Turkey Chili

Preparation Time: 15 Minutes

Cooking Time: 120 Minutes

Servings: 8

Ingredients:

- 2 tablespoons olive oil

- 1 small yellow onion, chopped

- 1 green bell pepper, seeded and chopped

- 4 garlic cloves, minced

- 1 jalapeño pepper, chopped

- 1 teaspoon dried thyme, crushed

- 2 tablespoons red chili powder

- 1 tablespoon ground cumin

- 2 pounds lean ground turkey

- 2 cups fresh tomatoes, chopped finely

- 2 ounces' sugar-free tomato paste

- 2 cups homemade chicken broth

- 1 cup of water

- Salt and ground black pepper, as required

- 1 cup cheddar cheese, shredded

Directions:

1. In a large Dutch oven, heat oil over medium heat and sauté the onion and bell pepper for about 5–7 minutes.

2. Add the garlic, jalapeño pepper, thyme, and spices and sauté for about 1 minute.

3. Add the turkey and cook for about 4–5 minutes.

4. Stir in the tomatoes, tomato paste, and cacao powder, and cook for about 2 minutes.

5. Add in the broth and water and bring to a boil.

6. Now, reduce the heat to low and simmer, covered for about 2 hours.

7. Add in salt and black pepper and remove from the heat.

8. Top with cheddar cheese and serve hot.

Nutrition: Calories 308, Fat 20, Carbs 10, Protein 8

CHAPTER 5:

Dinner Recipes

12.   Mussels in Red Wine Sauce

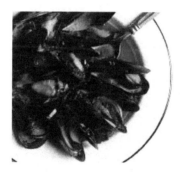

Preparation time: 5 minutes

Cooking time: 5 minutes

Servings: 2

Ingredients:

- 800g mussels

- 2 x 400g tins of chopped tomatoes

- 25g butter

- 1 fresh chives, chopped

- 1 fresh parsley, chopped

- 1 bird's-eye chili, finely chopped

- 4 cloves of garlic, crushed

- 400mls red wine Juice of 1 lemon

Directions:

1. Wash the mussels, remove their beards, and set them aside. Heat the butter in a large saucepan and add in the red wine. Reduce

the heat and add the parsley, chives, chili, and garlic whilst

stirring. Add in the tomatoes, lemon juice, and mussels. Cover

the saucepan and cook for 2-3. Remove the saucepan from the

heat and take out any mussels which haven't opened and discard

them. Serve and eat immediately.

Nutrition: calories: 364, carbs: 3.3, Fat: 4.9, Protein: 8

13.   Roast Balsamic Vegetables

Preparation time: 10 minutes

Cooking time: 45 minutes

Servings: 4

Ingredients:

- 4 tomatoes, chopped 2 red onions, chopped

- 3 sweet potatoes, peeled and chopped

- 100g red chicory (or if unavailable, use yellow)

- 100g kale, finely chopped

- 300g potatoes, peeled and chopped

- 5 stalks of celery, chopped

- 1 bird's-eye chili, de-seeded and finely chopped

- 2g fresh parsley, chopped

- 2gs fresh coriander (cilantro) chopped

- 3 teaspoons olive oil

- 2 teaspoons balsamic vinegar

- 1 teaspoon mustard Sea salt Freshly ground black pepper

Directions:

1. Place the olive oil, balsamic, mustard, parsley, and coriander (cilantro) into a bowl and mix well. Toss all the remaining ingredients into the dressing and season with salt and pepper. Transfer the vegetables to an ovenproof dish and cook in the oven at 200C/400F for 45 minutes.

Nutrition: Calories: 310, carbs: 1, Protein: 0.2g

14.   Tomato and Goat's Pizza

Preparation time: 15 minutes

Cooking time: 20 minutes

Servings: 2

Ingredients:

- 225g buckwheat flour

- 2 teaspoons dried yeast Pinch of salt

- 150mls slightly water 1 teaspoon olive oil

For the Topping:

- 75g feta cheese, crumbled

- 75g peseta (or tomato paste)

- 1 tomato, sliced 1 red onion, finely chopped

- 25g rocket (arugula) leaves, chopped

Directions:

1. In a bowl, combine all the ingredients for the pizza dough, then allow it to stand for at least an hour until it has doubled in size. Roll the dough out to a size to suit you. Spoon the passata onto the base and add the rest of the toppings. Bake in the oven at 200C/400F for 15-20 minutes or until browned at the edges and crispy and serve.

Nutrition: Calories: 585 carbs: 77 Fat: 8, Protein: 22.9

15.   Tender Spiced Lamb

Preparation time: 20 minutes

Cooking time: 4 hours 20 minutes

Servings: 8

Ingredients:

- 1.35kg lamb shoulder

- 3 red onions, sliced

- 3 cloves of garlic, crushed

- 1 bird's eye chili, finely chopped

- 1 teaspoon turmeric

- 1 teaspoon ground cumin

- ½ teaspoon ground coriander (cilantro)

- ¼ teaspoon ground cinnamon

Directions:

1. In a bowl, combine the chili, garlic, and spices with olive oil. Coat the lamb with the spice mixture and marinate it for an hour, or overnight if you can. Heat the remaining oil in a pan, add the lamb and brown it for 3-4 minutes on all sides to seal it. Place the lamb in an ovenproof dish. Add in the red onions and cover the dish with foil. Transfer to the oven and roast at 170C/325F for 4 hours. The lamb should be extremely tender and falling off the bone. Serve with rice or couscous, salad or vegetables.

Nutrition: calories: 455, carbs 28, Fat: 9.8 Protein: 20

16. Chili Cod Fillets

Preparation time: 10 minutes Cooking time: 10 minutes

Servings: 4

Ingredients:

- 4 cod fillets

- 2 teaspoons fresh parsley, chopped

- 2 bird's-eye chilies (or more if you like it hot)

- 2 cloves of garlic, chopped

- 4 teaspoons olive oil

Directions:

1. Heat olive oil in a frying pan, add the fish, and cook for 7-8

   minutes or until thoroughly cooked, turning once halfway

through. Remove and keep warm. Pour the remaining olive oil

into the pan and add the chili, chopped garlic, and parsley. Warm

it thoroughly. Serve the fish onto plates and pour the warm chili

oil over it.

Nutrition: calories: 246, carbs: 5, Fat: 0.5, Protein: 18

CHAPTER 6:

Soup and Salads

17.   Coconut Watercress Soup

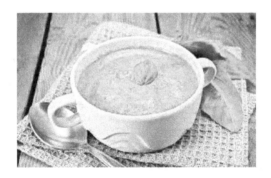

Preparation time: 10 minutes

Cooking time: 20 minutes

Servings: 4

Ingredients:

- 1 teaspoon coconut oil

- 1 onion, diced

- ¾ cup coconut milk

Directions:

1. Melt the coconut oil in a large pot over medium-high heat. Add the onion and cook until soft, about 5 minutes, then add the peas and the water. Bring to a boil, then lower the heat and add the watercress, mint, salt, and pepper.

2. Cover and simmer for 5 minutes. Stir in the coconut milk, and purée the soup until smooth in a blender or with an immersion blender.

3. Try this soup with any other fresh, leafy green—anything from spinach to collard greens to arugula to swiss chard.

Nutrition: calories 170, fat 3, carbs 18, protein 6

18.   Roasted Red Pepper and Butternut Squash Soup

Preparation time: 10 minutes

Cooking time: 45 minutes

Servings: 6

Ingredients:

- 1 small butternut squash

- 1 tablespoon olive oil

- 1 teaspoon sea salt

- 2 red bell peppers

- 1 yellow onion

- 1 head garlic

- 2 cups water, or vegetable broth

- Zest and juice of 1 lime

- 1 to 2 tablespoons tahini

- Pinch cayenne pepper

- ½ teaspoon ground coriander

- ½ teaspoon ground cumin

- Toasted squash seeds (optional)

Directions:

1. Preheat the oven to 350°f.

2. Prepare the squash for roasting by cutting it in half lengthwise, scooping out the seeds, and poking some holes in the flesh with a fork. Reserve the seeds if desired.

3. Rub a small amount of oil over the flesh and skin, then rub with a bit of sea salt and put the halves skin-side down in a large

baking dish. Put it in the oven while you prepare the rest of the vegetables.

4. Prepare the peppers the exact same way, except they do not need to be poked.

5. Slice the onion in half and rub oil on the exposed faces. Slice the top off the head of garlic and rub oil on the exposed flesh.

6. After the squash has cooked for 20 minutes, add the peppers, onion, and garlic, and roast for another 20 minutes. Optionally, you can toast the squash seeds by putting them in the oven in a separate baking dish 10 to 15 minutes before the vegetables are finished.

7. Keep a close eye on them. When the vegetables are cooked, take them out and let them cool before handling them. The squash will be very soft when poked with a fork.

8. Scoop the flesh out of the squash skin into a large pot (if you have an immersion blender) or into a blender.

9. Chop the pepper roughly, remove the onion skin and chop the onion roughly, and squeeze the garlic cloves out of the head, all into the pot or blender. Add the water, the lime zest and juice, and the tahini. Purée the soup, adding more water if you like, to your desired consistency. Season with the salt, cayenne, coriander, and cumin. Serve garnished with toasted squash seeds (if using).

Nutrition: calories 150, fat 3, carbs 20, protein 6

19.   Tomato Pumpkin Soup

Preparation time: 25 minutes

Cooking time: 15 minutes

Servings: 4

Ingredients:

- 2 cups pumpkin, diced

- 1/2 cup tomato, chopped

- 1/2 cup onion, chopped

- 1 1/2 tsp curry powder

- 1/2 tsp paprika

- 2 cups vegetable stock

- 1 tsp olive oil

- 1/2 tsp garlic, minced

Directions:

1. In a saucepan, add oil, garlic, and onion and sauté for 3 minutes over medium heat.

2. Add remaining ingredients into the saucepan and bring to a boil.

3. Reduce heat and cover, and simmer for 10 minutes.

4. Puree the soup using a blender until smooth.

5. Stir well and serve warm.

Nutrition: calories 70, fat 3, carbs 13, protein 1

CHAPTER 7:

Smoothie Recipes

20.   **Sweet Green Smoothie**

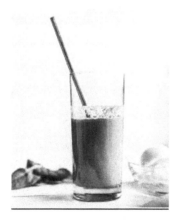

Preparation Time: 10 minutes

Cooking Time: 0 minutes

Servings: 1

Ingredients:

- 2 tablespoons flax seeds

- 1/2 cup wheatgrass

- 1 mango

- 1 cup pomegranate juice

Directions:

1. Add all ingredients to the blender and blend until smooth and creamy.

2. Serve immediately and enjoy.

Nutrition: calories 177, fat 1, carbs 21, protein 5

21.   Avocado Mango Smoothie

Preparation Time: 10 minutes

Cooking Time: 0 minutes

Servings: 2

Ingredients:

- 1 cup ice cubes

- 1/2 cup mango

- 1/2 avocado 1 tablespoon ginger

- 3 kale leaves 1 cup coconut water

Directions:

1. Toss in all your ingredients into your blender, then process until

   smooth.

2. Serve and Enjoy.

Nutrition: calories 290, fat 3, carbs 18, protein 11

22.   Super Healthy Green Smoothie

Preparation Time: 10 minutes

Cooking Time: 0 minutes

Servings: *2*

Ingredients:

- 1 teaspoon spirulina powder

- 1 cup coconut water

- 2 cups mixed greens

- 1 tablespoon ginger

- 4 tablespoon lemon juice

- 2 celery stalks

- 1 cup cucumber, chopped

- 1 green pear, core removed

- 1 banana

Directions:

1. Add all ingredients to the blender and blend until smooth and

   creamy.

2. Serve immediately and enjoy.

Nutrition: calories 161, fat 1, carbs 19, protein 7

23.   Spinach Coconut Smoothie

Preparation Time: 10 minutes

Cooking Time: 0 minutes

Servings: 2

Ingredients:

- 2 tablespoons unsweetened coconut flakes

- 2 cups fresh pineapple

- 1/2 cup coconut water

- 1 and 1/2 cups coconut milk 2 cups fresh spinach

Directions:

1. Add all ingredients to the blender and blend until smooth and

   creamy.

2. Serve immediately and enjoy.

Nutrition: calories 290, fat 1, carbs 22, protein 8

CHAPTER 8:

Fish and Seafood Recipes

24.   Baked Tuna 'Crab' Cakes

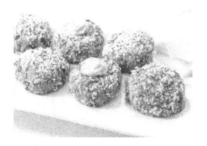

Preparation Time: 20 minutes

Cooking Time: 40 minutes

Servings: 4

Ingredients:

- 1 can chunk light tuna in water, drained and flaked

- 1 cup graham cracks crumbs

- 1 zucchini, shredded

- 1/2 green bell pepper, chopped

- 1/2 onion, finely chopped 1/2 cup green onions, chopped

- 2 cloves garlic, pressed or minced

- 1 teaspoon finely chopped jalapeno pepper

- 1/2 cup tofu

- 1/4 cup fat-free sour cream

- 1 lime, juiced

- 1 tablespoon dried basil

- 1 teaspoon ground black pepper

- 2 eggs

Directions:

1. Preheat oven to 350 degrees F. Line a baking sheet with aluminum foil, and spray with cooking spray.

2. Scoop up about ¼ cup of the tuna mixture and gently form it into a compact patty. And place the cakes onto the prepared baking sheet. Spray the tops of the cakes with cooking oil spray.

3. Bake in the preheated oven until the tops of the cakes are beginning to brown, about 20 minutes. Flip each cake, spray with cooking spray, and bake until the cakes are cooked through and lightly browned about 20 more minutes.

Nutrition: Calories 63, fat 24, carbs 18, Protein 35,

25.   Baked Fennel & Garlic Sea Bass

Preparation time: 5 minutes

Cooking time: 15 minutes

Servings: 2

Ingredients:

- 1 lemon

- ½ sliced fennel bulb

- 6 oz. sea bass fillets

- 1 tsp. black pepper

- 2 garlic cloves

Direction:

1. Preheat the oven to 375°F/Gas Mark 5.

2. Sprinkle black pepper over the Sea Bass.

3. Slice the fennel bulb and garlic cloves.

4. Add 1 salmon fillet and half the fennel and garlic to one sheet of baking paper or tin foil.

5. Squeeze in 1/2 lemon juices.

6. Repeat for the other fillet.

7. Fold and add to the oven for 12-15 minutes or until fish is thoroughly cooked through.

8. Meanwhile, add boiling water to your couscous, cover, and allow to steam.

9. Serve with your choice of rice or salad.

Nutrition: calories 221, fat 8, carbs 4, protein 14

26. Lemon, Garlic & Cilantro Tuna and Rice

Preparation time: 5 minutes

Cooking time: 0 minutes

Servings: 2

Ingredients:

- ½ cup arugula

- 1 tbsp. extra virgin olive oil

- 1 cup cooked rice

- 1 tsp. black pepper

- ¼ finely diced red onion

- 1 juiced lemon

- 3 oz. canned tuna

- 2 tbsps. Chopped fresh cilantro

Directions:

1. Mix the olive oil, pepper, cilantro, and red onion in a bowl.

2. Stir in the tuna, cover, and leave in the fridge for as long as possible (if you can), or serve immediately.

3. When ready to eat, serve up with the cooked rice and arugula!

Nutrition: calories 320, fat 7, carbs 3, protein 42

27.   Cod & Green Bean Risotto

Preparation time: 4 minutes

Cooking time: 40 minutes

Servings: 2

Ingredients:

- ½ cup arugula

- 1 finely diced white onion

- 4 oz. cod fillet

- 1 cup white rice

- 2 lemon wedges

- 1 cup boiling water

- ¼ tsp. black pepper

- 1 cup low sodium chicken broth

- 1 tbsp. extra virgin olive oil

- ½ cup green beans

Directions:

1. Heat the oil in a large pan on medium heat.

2. Sauté the chopped onion for 5 minutes until soft before adding in the rice and stirring for 1-2 minutes.

3. Combine the broth with boiling water.

4. Add half of the liquid to the pan and stir slowly.

5. Slowly add the rest of the liquid whilst continuously stirring for up to 20-30 minutes.

6. Stir in the green beans to the risotto.

7. Place the fish on top of the rice, cover, and steam for 10 minutes.

8. Ensure the water does not dry out and keep topping up until the rice is cooked thoroughly.

9. Use your fork to break up the fish fillets and stir into the rice.

10. Sprinkle with freshly ground pepper to serve and a squeeze of fresh lemon.

11. Garnish with the lemon wedges and serve with the arugula.

Nutrition: calories 219, fat 18, carbs 3, protein 40

28.   Sardine Fish Cakes

Preparation Time: 10 minutes

Cooking Time: 10 minutes

Servings: 4

Ingredients:

- 11 oz sardines, canned, drained

- 1/3 cup shallot, chopped

- 1 teaspoon chili flakes

- ½ teaspoon salt

- 2 tablespoon wheat flour, whole grain

- 1 egg, beaten

- 1 tablespoon chives, chopped

- 1 teaspoon olive oil

- 1 teaspoon butter

Directions:

1. Put the butter in the skillet and melt it.

2. Add shallot and cook it until translucent.

3. After this, transfer the shallot to the mixing bowl.

4. Add sardines, chili flakes, salt, flour, egg, chives, and mix up until smooth with the help of the fork.

5. Make the medium size cakes and place them in the skillet.

6. Add olive oil.

7. Roast the fish cakes for 3 minutes from each side over medium heat.

8. Dry the cooked fish cakes with a paper towel if needed and transfer to the serving plates.

Nutrition: calories 356, fat 23, carbs 1, protein 38

CHAPTER 9:

Poultry Recipes

29.   Sweet and Spicy Firecracker Chicken

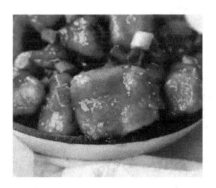

Preparation time: 9 minutes

Cooking Time: 35 minutes

Servings: 4

Ingredients:

- 1/2 cup packed light brown sugar

- 1/3 cup buffalo sauce

- 1 tablespoon apple cider vinegar

- salt

- 1/4 teaspoon red pepper flakes

- 1 lb. boneless skinless chicken breast

- 1/2 cup cornstarch

- 2 large eggs

Directions:

1. Start by cutting the chicken breast into 1-inch cubes.

2. Mix buffalo sauce in a bowl, apple cider vinegar, salt, and red pepper flakes.

3. Place the cornstarch in a plastic container or bag.

4. Beat the eggs in a bowl.

5. Toss the chicken in the cornstarch, then dip it in the egg.

6. Cook chicken in your air fryer at 360F for about 5 minutes; the chicken does not need to be fully cooked, only crisp on the outside.

7. Place the chicken in a baking pan and pour the buffalo sauce mixture over it. Return to the air fryer.

8. Continue to bake at 350F for 30 minutes.

Nutrition: Calories: 385, Fat: 7, Carbs: 38, Protein: 40

30.   Fried Chicken Livers

Preparation time: 9 minutes

Cooking Time: 10 minutes

Servings: 4

Ingredients:

- 1 lb. chicken livers

- 1 cup flour

- 1/2 cup cornmeal

- 2 teaspoons herbs Provence

- 3 eggs

- 2 tablespoons milk

Directions:

1. Clean and rinse the livers, pat dry.

2. Beat eggs in a shallow bowl and mix in milk.

3. In another bowl, combine flour, cornmeal, and seasoning, mixing until even.

4. Dip the livers in the egg mix, then toss them in the flour mix.

5. Air fry at 375F for 10 minutes. Toss at least once halfway through.

Nutrition: Calories: 409, Fat: 11, Carbs: 37, Protein: 36

31.   Turkey with Maple Mustard Glaze

Preparation time: 13 minutes

Cooking Time: minutes

Servings: 4

Ingredients:

- 2 teaspoons olive oil

- 3 lbs. whole turkey breast

- 1 teaspoon dried thyme

- 1/2 teaspoon dried sage

- 1/2 teaspoon smoked paprika

- 1 teaspoon salt

- 1/2 teaspoon black pepper

- 1/4 cup maple syrup

- 2 tablespoons Dijon mustard

- 1 tablespoon butter

Directions:

1. Preheat the air fryer to 350°F. Brush the entire turkey breast with olive oil.

2. Combine dry seasonings and toss to mix.

3. Rub the seasonings over the turkey and put it in the air fryer, frying for 25 minutes.

4. Turn it on one side and fry for another 12 minutes. Turn it on the other side, then cook for 11 more minutes.

5. Melt the butter in a bowl and mix in syrup and mustard.

6. Return the turkey to its upright position and brush the syrup mix over the turkey.

7. Cook for 5 more minutes before serving. Enjoy!!

Nutrition: Calories: 404, Fat: 8, Carbs: 14, Protein: 58

32. Chicken Parmesan

Preparation time: 9 minutes

Cooking Time: 10 minutes

Servings: 4

Ingredients:

- 2 (8 ounce) chicken breast

- 6 tablespoons seasoned breadcrumbs

- 2 tablespoons parmesan cheese

- 1 tablespoon olive oil

- 6 tablespoons mozzarella cheese

- 1/2 cup marinara sauce

- Cooking spray

Directions:

1. Cut the chicken in half vertically to create 4 breasts.

2. Mix the breadcrumbs and parmesan together in a bowl.

3. Brush the chicken with olive oil.

4. Press the chicken into the breadcrumb mix.

5. Preheat the air fryer to 360°F.

6. Place 2 chicken breasts in the basket and spray with cooking spray.

7. Cook for 6 minutes.

8. Flip the chicken and top with 1 tablespoon marinara and 1 - 1/2 tablespoons mozzarella.

9. Cook for 3 more minutes, then repeat with the other 2 breasts.

Nutrition: Calories: 250, Fat: 14, Carbs: 11, Protein: 18

CHAPTER 10:

Vegan & Vegetarian

33.   Vegan Pear and Cranberry Cake

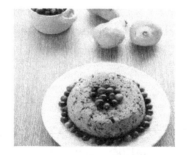

Preparation time: 5 minutes

Cooking Time: 45 minutes

Servings: 4-6

Ingredients:

- 1 1/4 cup whole wheat pastry flour

- 1/8 teaspoon sea salt

- baking powder

- baking soda

- 1/2 teaspoon ground cardamom

- Cup of halved unsweetened nondairy milk

- 2 tablespoons coconut oil

- 2 tablespoons ground flax seeds

- 1/4 cup agave

- 2 cups water

- Cup of halved chopped cranberries

- 1 cup chopped pear

Directions:

1. Grease a Bundt pan; set aside.

2. In a mixing, mix all dry ingredients together. In another bowl, mix all wet ingredients; whisk the wet ingredients into the dry until smooth.

3. Fold in the add-ins and spread the mixture into the pan; cover with foil.

4. Place pan in your air fryer toast oven and add water in the bottom and bake at 370 degrees F for 35 minutes.

5. When done, use a toothpick to check for doneness. If it comes out clean, then the cake is ready, if not, bake for 5-10 more minutes, checking frequently to avoid burning.

6. Remove the cake and let stand for 10 minutes before transferring from the pan.

7. Enjoy!

Nutrition: Calories 309, Carbs 14, Fat 27, Protein 22

34.   Oven Steamed Broccoli

Preparation time: 8 minutes

Cooking Time: 3 minutes

Servings: 2

Ingredients:

- 1 pound broccoli florets

- 1½ cups water

- Salt and pepper to taste

- I tsp. extra virgin olive oil

Directions:

1. Add water to the bottom of your air fryer toast oven and set the

   basket on top.

2. Toss the broccoli florets with salt pepper, and olive oil until evenly combined, then transfer to the basket of your air fryer toast oven.

3. Cook at 350 degrees for 5 minutes.

4. Remove the basket and serve the broccoli.

Nutrition: Calories 160, Fat 12, Carbs 6, Protein 13

35.   Brussels sprouts

Preparation time: 11 minutes **Cooking Time**: 13 minutes

Servings: 4

Ingredients:

- 2 pound Brussels sprouts, halved

- 1 tbsp. chopped almonds

- 1 tbsp. rice vinegar

- 2 tbsp. sriracha sauce

- 1/4 cup gluten-free soy sauce

- 2 tbsp. sesame oil

- 1/2 tbsp. cayenne pepper

- 1 tbsp. smoked paprika

- 1 tsp. onion powder

- 2 tsp. garlic powder

- 1 tsp. red pepper flakes

- Salt and pepper

Directions:

1. Preheat your air fryer toast oven to 370 degrees F.

2. Meanwhile, place your air fryer toast oven's pan on medium heat and cook the almonds for 3 minutes, then add in all the remaining ingredients.

3. Place the pan in the air fryer toast oven and cook for 8-10 minutes or until done to desire. Serve hot over a bed of steamed rice. Enjoy!

Nutrition: Calories 216, Fat 18, Carbs 9, Protein 18

36. Power Roasted Roots Soup

Preparation time: 18 minutes

Cooking Time: 1 hour

Servings: 5

Ingredients:

- 2 tablespoons extra virgin olive oil

- 2 red onions, quartered

- 2 red peppers, deseeded, chopped

- 3 tomatoes, halved

- 3 carrots, peeled, diced

- 2 sweet potatoes, peeled, diced

- 2 cans light coconut milk

- 1 teaspoon ground cumin

- 1 tablespoon smoked paprika, plus extra for garnish

- 2 inches fresh root ginger, peeled, minced

- 1 bay leaf

- Salt and black pepper

- Chopped coriander to garnish

- Lime wedges

Directions

1. Preheat oven your air fryer toast oven to 400°F.

2. In your air fryer toast oven's pan, mix all the veggies and oil and roast in the air fryer toast oven for about 40 minutes or until cooked.

3. Remove from air fryer toast oven.

4. Chop the roasted vegetables and place them in a saucepan; add the remaining ingredients and stir to mix well; season with salt and bring the mixture to a gentle boil in a saucepan and then simmer for about 20 minutes.

5. Divide the soup among six serving bowls and sprinkle each with coriander, black pepper, and smoked paprika.

6. Garnish with lime wedges and enjoy!

Nutrition: Calories 390, Carbs11, Fat 22, Protein 19

CHAPTER 11:

Pork recipes

37.   Pork Tenderloin

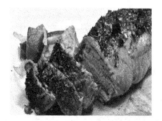

Preparation Time: 10 minutes

Cooking Time: 25 minutes

Servings: 4

Ingredients

- 1.5 lb. pork tenderloin

- 1 tbsp. olive oil

- 1/4 tsp. garlic powder

- 1/4 tsp. salt

Directions

1. Brine the tenderloin according to brining instructions, and this is optional. Take tenderloin out from the fridge 20 minutes before cooking. If it was brined, discard brine and rinse pork. Cut silver skin according to these given instructions.

2. Preheat air fryer toaster oven to 450F. In a bowl, mix olive oil, black pepper, and garlic powder. Add the salt If you did not brine the pork. Stir. Brush olive oil mixture all over tenderloin.

Put tenderloin in the air fryer tray, bending it if needed for it to fit. Cook it for 10 minutes, or until it has reached the desired doneness as indicated on an instant-read thermometer, 145-160F has been recommended by the US Pork Board. This will take 8 to 15 extra minutes. Set aside for at least 5 minutes before slicing into 1/2 to 3/4 inch pieces. Serve immediately.

Nutrition: calories 321, fat 28, carbs 7, protein 42

38.   Quick Pork Belly

Preparation Time: 20 minutes

Cooking Time: 65 minutes

Servings: 4

Ingredients

- 2 lb. piece of pork belly

- Olive oil spray

- Salt

Directions

1. Take out the pork belly, if you are using a packaged piece of pork belly, then there is no need to dry the skin.

2. Score the skin with a sharp knife by slicing the rind and taking care not to cut through to the meat underneath.

3. Put on the tray inside your air fryer toaster oven, rind side up. Spray equally with olive oil cooking spray.

4. Cover it equally and thickly with a layer of cracked salt. Set your air fryer toaster oven to 180C for 45 minutes, then check the pork belly, if you see one side cooking faster than the other, it can be a good idea to flip the rack 180 degrees.

5. Now turn the air fryer up to full (230C) and set more 15 minutes. Some pieces of pork will be ready after these steps, others might need more than 15 minutes. Your pork belly will be done when the crackling is hard and crispy.

6. Different air fryers can have their own cooking times, so be aware of this when making your pork belly. Some air fryers toaster oven may require more or less cooking time.

Nutrition: calories 390, fat 20, carbs 3, protein 34

CHAPTER 12:

Snack Recipes

39. Roasted Zucchini Boats with Ground Beef

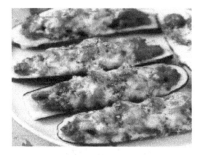

Preparation Time: 15 minutes

Cooking Time: 35 minutes

Servings: 8

Ingredients:

- Cooking spray

- 4 medium zucchinis

- 1 tablespoon olive oil

- 4 ounces cremini mushrooms, diced

- 2 garlic cloves, minced 8 ounces 90% lean ground beef

- ½ cup jarred tomato sauce

- ¼ teaspoon salt ⅛ teaspoon freshly ground black pepper

- ½ cup shredded part-skim mozzarella cheese

Directions:

1. Preheat the oven to 350°F. Coat a baking dish with cooking spray. Halve the zucchini lengthwise and, using a teaspoon,

scoop out the seeds. Place the zucchini in the baking pan, leaving space between each zucchini.

2. In a large sauté pan or skillet over medium heat, heat the olive oil. Add the mushrooms and sauté until softened. Mix in garlic and cook until translucent.

3. Add the ground beef and cook for 5 minutes, until browned, breaking up the pieces. Add the tomato sauce, salt, and pepper, and stir to combine. Continue until totally cooked. Let it cool for about 10 minutes.

4. Spoon 2 heaping tablespoons of beef mixture into each zucchini boat, and top each boat with 1 tablespoon of shredded mozzarella. Bake until it's cook.

Nutrition: calories 197, fat 5, carbs 4, protein 9

CHAPTER 13:

Appetizer Recipes

40.   Salmon Burger

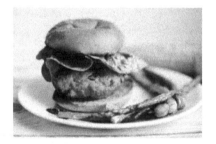

Preparation Time: 15 minutes

Cooking Time: 15 minutes

Servings: 6

Ingredients:

- 16 ounces (450 g) pink salmon, minced

- 1 cup (250 g) prepared mashed potatoes

- 1 medium (110 g) onion, chopped

- 1 stalk celery (about 60 g), finely chopped 1 large egg (about 60 g), lightly beaten

- 2 tablespoons (7 g) fresh cilantro, chopped 1 cup (100 g) breadcrumbs

- Vegetable oil, for deep frying alt and freshly ground black pepper

Directions:

1. Combine the salmon, mashed potatoes, onion, celery, egg, and cilantro in a mixing bowl. Season to taste and mix thoroughly.

Spoon about 2 Tablespoon mixture, roll in breadcrumbs, and then form into small patties.

2. Heat oil in non-stick frying pan. Cook your salmon patties for 5 minutes on each side or until golden brown and crispy.

3. Serve in burger buns and with coleslaw on the side if desired.

Nutrition: calories 230, Fat 7, Carbs 20, Protein 18

Conclusion

When you desire a structure and need to rapidly lose weight, the present diet is the perfect solution.

Its extremely low calories eating plans of the optavia diet will definitely help you to shed more pounds

Before you start any meal replacement diet plan, carefully consider if truly it possible for you to continue with a specific diet plan

When you have decided to stick with this regimen and make progress with your weight loss goal, ensure you have a brilliant knowledge about optimal health management to enable and archive the desired result effortlessly in the shortest period of time.

CPSIA information can be obtained
at www.ICGtesting.com
Printed in the USA
BVHW062328150621
609638BV00012B/997